ALWAYS SUBLIME, NEVER RIDICULOUS

by
Sharon Rose

**Five years on, author of
Single Salsa Survivor:
The Journal of a Breast-Cancer Survivor**

ARTHUR H. STOCKWELL LTD
Torrs Park, Ilfracombe, Devon, EX34 8BA
Established 1898
www.ahstockwell.co.uk

British Library Cataloguing-in-Publication Data.
A catalogue record for this book is available
from the British Library.

By the same author:
Single Salsa Survivor
Living in Grief, Loving in Grief

This book is dedicated to my mum,
Sheila, on her 80th birthday, 11 May 2014.
Thank you for your inspiration through your love, strength
and loyalty. Happy birthday to the best mum in the world.

ISBN 978-0-7223-4249-7
Printed in Great Britain by
Arthur H. Stockwell Ltd
Torrs Park   Ilfracombe
Devon EX34 8BA

Introduction

At last I feel happy about how my third book has evolved. I had thoughts about writing solely about my recent experience on benefits and my struggles with money and calling it *The Sublime to the Ridiculous*. That experience deserves a chapter that could help stimulate thought and reflection about attitudes to money; but I couldn't write a book whining about not having money when I live in the luxury of the UK and children in third-world countries are dying of pneumonia and gastric infections caused by dirty water. The period of my life some might call ridiculous actually provided me and my family with lifelong skills on money management and prioritizing, and it gave us a very interesting lesson on how to live, love and laugh on fresh air.

Five years ago in 2005–6 I was starting my cancer treatment; my life had changed in a whirlwind; plans had faded into fear – fear of dying. I went into fighting mode to live. My lifelong goal and my short-term goal were the same: to stay *alive*. I had no crystal ball, no psychic insight into the future, no guarantee that I would live or die. Uncertainty ruled my brain.

Here and Now, The Past, The Present and All That Happened In Between

It's 22 February 2011, I am at my five-year health check at the hospital, and I have that same sense of anticipation, of not knowing what will happen. The thought of it gives me butterflies in my tummy – or perhaps they should be called 'fear flies'! Fear again! It is one of those momentous times when within one day your life can change dramatically, for better or worse. Emotional and psychological balls are juggled in the air. Everything depends on how the conversation begins. Will it be "Well, I am pleased to say . . ." or "I am sorry to say that . . ."?

Women are coming in and out of the scan room and going home and I am still sitting here. Fear grips me again like a knife of déjà vu. Check-ups are like checkouts to people in remission with cancer, every blood test is a minefield and our bodies are saturated with adrenalin.

Something always manages to slip into my mind to create a smile. I remember crying uncontrollably in my dentist's waiting room – I had to be taken into a side room, and the receptionist was wondering what had happened. It was the first X-ray I had a after my cancer treatment: an X-ray of my jaw because I had a painful clicking jaw. Ouch! The result showed that it was not jaw cancer, as I had thought, but over-usage of the jaw muscle caused by chewing gum. Chewing gum was an occupational hazard of salsa dancing because the close proximity of other dancers meant that smelly breath was not an option. In the early days after treatment my friend Jill would listen to me as I went into panic mode, imagining that every pain was the cancer returning. I would have cancer of every part of my anatomy until in the end I jokingly told Jill that, judging by the way I was

4

hysterical about every pain, I must have the worst ever case of cancer of the personality.

Over time the fear fades a little, especially when you have a cough or a cold that you actually recover from.

Today is different. I am still waiting in the waiting area, and I am called back to the familiar sight of sombre faces. I start planning in my head that future again – or should I say the end of my future? What about Erica? I have to live a lot more years now than I did last time: Lisa was fourteen and I had to get to eighteen if I could, but Erica is only four years of age. I am scared now.

The dreaded sentences echo in my head: "I am sorry to say that we have found a shadow – a suspicious area in your left breast. We are going to scan right now."

I lie on the couch rocketed to cancer planet in a second, only to jump out of the rocket with a parachute, floating on the words "Well, I am pleased to say that everything looks OK."

And so continues the life of Sharon Rose, from avalanche to still waters, from thunderstorms to sunshine and soft sand.

I walk out of the hospital having learnt one valuable lesson: whilst I live and breathe my life will not stand still. I sit in the car and contemplate how lucky I am.

I look at my mum and feel enormous sorrow for the pressure she must be under. She is always with me on my roller coaster of life.

I know a little girl who is going to get the biggest hug ever as soon as I get home.

But that is not what this story is about. This story is about yesterday and the whole five years I have been granted to live my life to the full. It is not about what tomorrow brings – that is another story.

It took me at least three years to plan tomorrow. Only after cognitive behaviour therapy did I manage to see that whilst I am on this earth I have to make the best of life and I learnt that achieving even small goals would lift my mood. These small achievements were moving me out of the morbid comfortable cancer zone, and I knew I would be forgiven by people for my insecurities and my impulsive behaviour. But progress was slow. It takes time to fit back into society. People begin to forget your illness as you begin to look well and healthy, and even your own memories fade. All of a sudden trivia raises its head and you moan about the weather; you start to put off today what you can do tomorrow. After five years had gone by I realised I had been granted a second chance in life. I had unfinished business. The last five years had been far from uneventful, thanks to the escapades of my first born.

Fiona

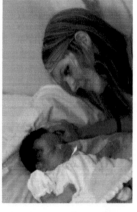

My daughter, Fiona, aged now twenty-six years, came into my bed in the morning like old times, and as we talked and talked it was evident that our mother–daughter bond was strong despite the traumatic, emotionally stressful times we had been through in the last five years.

For the first time in five years my daughter was in reach again, and as we talked like old times we laughed at silly jokes that only we two understand. We finally talked about how and why our relationship had improved so much in recent months. Erica (Fiona's daughter, now aged four) had been asking questions about why she didn't live with her own mummy. The work excuse was wearing thin, and we talked about in time telling Erica about her mum's difficulties. I had my worries that Erica would start blaming herself, as children sometimes do when they do not understand the Mummy-and-Daddy dynamics in whatever situation – whether separation or divorce of parents, or the situation that Fiona and I found ourselves.

Erica four years ago was seen as a gift to all the family, and she is. Fiona is stunning and beautiful, and she has happily in the last few years spent some time as a lap dancer/pole dancer.

She reiterated to me that she loved her job. She said she was born to shine, to be on stage, to dance, to wear beautiful dresses, to be admired. I had come to terms with Fiona's lifestyle. Before, my perception of what I thought was the right way was not how Fiona saw it. She always used to say her body was her tool for working, and that's why she had to spend money looking good; nail salons, spray tans and hair extensions were her priority. This was alien to me. I had always washed my face with Fairy soap and washed my hair in Vosene.

When my brother Adrian took his own life he was a lonely unemployed musician of amazing talent. His death made me question my own stereotypical views on what is the norm. I loved the art world, encouraging my children in their individual vocational dreams, but I didn't do enough to make Adrian feel important and proud of his talent when he was alive.

Fiona is a pole dancer. I now accept and respect her for her own choice regarding what she does to earn her own money, and I have stopped focusing on how it affects me and worrying about what people think of me. Honestly, I would never criticise this profession – I have never seen a newspaper clipping, or heard derogatory comments about the men who frequent pole-dancing clubs.

Fiona in Selfridge's

I didn't really understand Fiona's personality until 13 February 2011. I booked, as a surprise for Valentine's Day, tickets for the Valentine's weekend showing at the oldest cinema in Birmingham to see *Breakfast at Tiffany's* starring the beautiful Audrey Hepburn and the very handsome George Peppard. But I saw more than a movie that day – I saw Audrey Hepburn play a part that replicated my own daughter's life as an adult. The flighty, self-absorbed character in the film could not find attachment easily, and focused on money because having it replaced love and attention and helped with the fantasy world she lived in. The cat had no name, but she had many because she couldn't find one she was comfortable with. The best line in the film was spoken by the affectionate male friend of Holly Golightly: "Yes, she is a phony, but she is a real phony."

Fiona wasn't actually a glamour model, or a wag, or a pop star, but she looked like a glamour model, she sang like a pop star, and she made sure she dated footballers. She was born to shine.

Fiona would have been best placed in the 1950s when women looked beautiful day and night, wore designer clothes, and diamonds were a girl's best friend. And so for me *Breakfast at Tiffany's* became Fiona in Selfridge's.

Fiona and I talked and she reflected on her difficulties. She told me how what comes naturally to most people (for example, turn-taking in conversation, empathy and the ability to assess moods and situations) takes a great effort for her. Fiona is working out every minute what life really means and what is going on in the world around her, and this can be a mentally draining task. She told me how sustained eye contact with people she knows well makes her feel uncomfortable. Eye contact is the window through which we know what other people are thinking. Sustained eye contact between men and women is one of the clues that tell us we have chemistry with someone of the opposite sex. Fiona explains that this helps her detach herself from the men she meets in her job as a lap dancer.

I had learnt not to comfort Fiona with hugs or other physical contact as this made her feel uncomfortable. I had come to accept all her quirky ways, because challenging them was impossible without a follow-through of meltdowns and fallings-out and emotional upset for both of us. I only challenged her behaviour if I felt she compromised others. I had learnt to accept rather than to try to change and cure.

Over the years there have been times when Fiona would function really well and I in particular would be lulled into a false sense of security. We tried letting her have unsupervised contact with Erica on numerous occasions when Fiona decided she could manage it, but these times lasted only two or three weeks at the most. On one occasion Fiona called me screaming and saying she had had to rugby tackle Erica, who had run off while they were in the park together. She called paramedics to the park because Erica had bumped her head. Fiona does make a drama out of a crisis. As an adult she does get into scrapes, and I am usually the first person she contacts.

I had to take parental responsibility for Erica, and in the end I decided supervised contact was the only option for the future. When Erica grew that little bit more and became more independent it became easier, and Fiona would have quality time taking Erica to the pictures.

Erica knows Fiona is her mum, and she understands she has difficulties, but above everything she loves her mum; and Fiona undoubtedly, in her own way, loves Erica.

My life changed from the minute I had Erica, and I have never had one regret, though sometimes I have felt guilty for receiving the love that a child normally reserves for his or her parents. I had Erica's unconditional love, but I was a single parent and loneliness sometimes put me into depths of despair. I was forty-six and most men struggled to come to terms with my cancer, let alone with the fact that I had a young child to care for. The men I met were on their second wind of freedom in life. But that's another story.

How Did We Get Here?

It seems an eternity since the day Fiona and I just turned up at the community mental-health services because I was so worried about my daughter's lifestyle and mental-health status. I cried and cried in desperation, and in the end Fiona was sent home – she appeared to be the more stable of us both, and I ended up being assessed and treated. My daughter's mental health is so fragile, but mine is too. It hit me like a thunderbolt that I don't know how to help my daughter as an adult. This is when I finally asked for help and started a course of cognitive behaviour therapy.

The Days When I Could I Protect My Child

Fiona's difficulties didn't become evident to me until the age of seven. Up until then I had an only child whom I adored and loved. There was very little need for two-way love – I loved her unconditionally and didn't notice anything unusual about her development. For a while I believed that life events were to blame for the little oddities of character that began to develop. There was a change in behaviour, with regular temper tantrums. She would scream and shout if I called her a big girl and not a little girl, and one day she ran off because she hated the smell of fruit gums. If I wanted to punish Fiona, then I would send her out to play with children her own age – Fiona's worst nightmare was when we were out with friends and I would insist she went to play. She would rather be attached to my hip.

Fiona spent hours in her bedroom singing at the top of her voice, in tune and with lyrics perfect. Singing was her haven; it enabled her to connect with emotion.

I moved her to a small village school. In her first primary school Fiona had struggled socially. She spent playtimes walking around and around the playground, never playing with friends. There were only six girls in her class at the village school and she survived primary school with little problem.

At home was different. I cannot remember everything that caused me concern, but I do remember that she required a lot of my attention. There were some associated problems with the muscles of her eyes and hyper-mobility of her joints, which made her clumsy and she needed physiotherapy. She used to rock against the settee, and she twitched and flapped her hands. I just thought Fiona was Fiona.

Her stepdad had very little tolerance, and for a time I didn't know whether Fiona's early childhood experience of family dysfunction had caused her sometimes challenging behaviour. The thought made me feel guilty. In one year, from 1989 to 1990, Fiona had to deal with the arrival of a new baby brother, and with a mum with depression – I say 'depression' rather than 'post-natal depression'. Life events for me were traumatic in that year. Previous to that I had had five miscarriages, so this pregnancy was precious. Problems started to snowball when I went into premature labour at twenty-six weeks. The medication to stop the labour affected my chronic heart condition and I nearly died. My husband was detaching himself from me, and during my traumatic labour a medical student held my hand. My husband cut himself off from his family until, four months later, I left with the two children and black plastic bags, to live with my sister-in-law and her husband (to whom I will be eternally grateful). We moved house and within a few months I met my second husband – vulnerable me! – and Fiona had to accept a new man in my life. Initially he appeared to be the perfect father, and to Ali and Lisa he was, but over the years I learnt to hate him for his nasty snide comments and after fifteen years I had had enough.

Fiona would never pick up on tension or mood changes in people and would continue in her own way, either laughing hysterically or shouting madly at inappropriate times. I would warn her every time not to swear when we went to Nanny's, but she took no notice. On one occasion when I was in the doctor's surgery seeing the paediatrician Fiona became impatient and fed up and started to sing at the top of her voice in the waiting room. Sometimes her character did make me laugh out loud! That is something Fiona and I have shared for years: a sense of humour. I admit to being quirky and eccentric myself – something I inherited from my dad.

Fiona didn't like holidays. She hated the texture of sand and, most of all, the change in routine.

I have regrets because as a mum I thought I could help her, change her, cure her; I floundered sometimes throughout her childhood because I didn't know what to do to help her.

I paid a £100 for an assessment for dyslexia at a time when dyslexia was also not recognised at all in health or education. The mental-health service for children and adolescents had a waiting list of about twelve months. Working in the health profession, I can see that there has been much progress in the service for children, though it is still a second-class service with long waiting lists and staff stretched to the limit. The government have at last recognised the need to promote health and prevent disease by investing in public health initiatives and providing more health visitors. At last there is some monetary investment from the government and there is a realisation that how we are bought up as babies and as young children has an enormous influence on our future lives. Our social and environmental experiences also affect our long-term holistic health.

Having a child that didn't fit in with the stereotypical norm gave me the experience to understand how other parents feel when their precious child is diagnosed with a condition that makes them different from their siblings or their peers. A grief process has to be followed in order to reach the final acceptance that such children need their parents' love unconditionally, as every child does. The outside world might find it difficult to understand them, so there is a risk that they will become isolated, creating more problems with the child's emotional well-being.

The diagnosis benefits the parents as much as it does the child. When finally there is no doubt, after a multidisciplinary assessment, that the child has a diagnostic condition there is relief for the parents. Up until that point it is not unusual for them to feel complete failures as parents because they aren't able to cure their child's disability. Physical disability is usually something the parent, the doctor and the world can see, but the autistic child, especially a 'high-functioning' child can look completely normal to the outside world. All the outside world can see is a child or adult behaving badly, and then come the critical looks and the condemnation. We had an appointment for an assessment to determine social communication difficulties, but we never got there. Why?

Secondary school had positives for Fiona. The passion in the music department led by an amazing music teacher encouraged Fiona to develop her singing talent. On the negative side, her developing beauty gave her a lot of male attention. In Fiona's end-of-school diary there were many derogatory comments and sexual references. I ripped it up and threw it away.

Fiona in her early teenage years had two very successful relationships with very nice older men, and for a while Fiona's life took a turn for the better and I had a rest from the caring role. However, when I was in hospital having my mastectomy Fiona needed attention and comfort. She found it, but not from me. I couldn't give her the comfort she needed. Nine months later, a week after my radiotherapy treatment finished, I was the birthing partner for Fiona, and Erica Lisa Angel Gilbert came into this world. This was a celebration of the gift of life – for Fiona a miracle and a gift for me! The pregnancy allowed her to escape the reality of her Mum having cancer. She now had another focus.

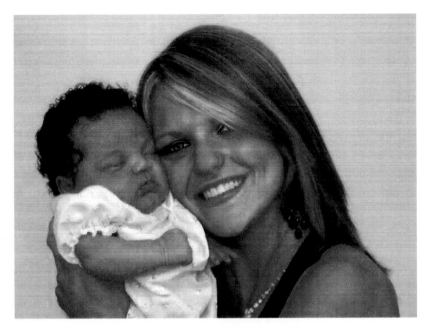

Fiona and Erica.
If Fiona had a crystal ball, maybe her smile would not
have been so bright.

There is a moral to this story: never judge a book by its cover. When making judgements we should make sure we have all the facts. But the most important thing of all is to embrace your children for the individuals they are. Love them unconditionally. You as the parent will be the only one who does.

The grief from my cancer experience was compounded by the fact that Fiona was struggling to cope with parenting and the unhappiness caused by her relationship breakdown. Whatever Fiona's personality traits, something affected her bonding with Erica and her ability to parent.

My philosophy is to celebrate life and live life to the full. I am so grateful to have seen Christmas again and I feel so very guilty about the way I felt. I took to my bed for two weeks over the Christmas period and watched *Holiday*, the romantic film, repeatedly. I laughed to myself at some silly sitcom, on my own.

I have come a long way since October, when I typed my first book, *Single Salsa Survivor*, at a hotel in the Lake District. I was with my salsa friends, writing in the day in the most enchanting, peaceful surroundings then livening up in the evening and dancing the night away. A memorable time! We called in at Blackpool to see the Christmas lights. Life was such fun then.

My new love interest of the moment agreed to help me with the presentation of my journal – put it together, ready to give to my closest family and friends as a tribute to them for helping me through my recent experience of breast cancer. I was naive enough to think a casual relationship was just a date in jeans, but I believe that even casual relationships could develop into love and marriage. I am such a dreamer sometimes! When he met someone else, and I was replaced and dumped, he expected me to accept the fact with a smile because, of course, I forgot, oh yes, our relationship was 'casual'. I am left with my completed journal that he so nicely typed for me; but my heart was broken and my pride bruised.

What kept me going and pulled me through the very lonely experience again was the precious quality time I spent with Erica – the walks by the river, saying hello to passers-by walking their dogs, feeding the ducks, singing all the good old, forever famous nursery rhymes. I loved the simplicity of Fridays: the park, the sunshine, the reward of Erica's smile. My love and attention was all that Erica and I needed.

Money is getting tighter and tighter and I am desperate to find time to 'grieve for my own mortality', but since the diagnosis of breast cancer there have been so many other complications in my life that I didn't have time – or didn't make time, that was more the problem.

For Christmas 2007 everyone, even the children, received a copy of my journal and a CD of my favourite songs – the ones that had reached my soul when I listened to the words during the most emotional time during cancer treatment. Christmas is definitely not about what you get as presents from other people; Christmas is about shopping, buying presents for loved ones and friends, getting caught up in the rush, running from shop to shop to get out of the cold . . . In fact, if you are really lucky, Christmas entails tramping in thick snow, listening to the subtle tones of Bing Crosby's 'White Christmas' and Wizard's 'I Wish It Could Be Christmas Every Day'.

But I didn't even enjoy Christmas this year. I let myself become self-absorbed with pity, though I am lucky to be alive for another Christmas. I have been physically, mentally, and emotionally saturated in sadness. Fiona is struggling to cope with Erica, and I am struggling to come to terms with the fact I have just got over cancer treatment. I am stranded in a whirlpool of emotions, trying to come to terms with the new me.

Fiona can't cope with parenting, and I am one step ahead: it is frighteningly obvious to me that it could mean Erica has to go into foster care. I cannot bear the thought.

I went to stay with Fiona for a month to try to keep Erica with her mum, but I could see that Fiona's attachment to Erica was decreasing. She never heard her cry in the night. I was helpless to stop the spiral of family dysfunction, and that included the effect on the two teenagers I had left at home. They had just had to struggle to come to terms with their mum having cancer; they had seen her fight for her life, and they had all brushed with the mortality issue, trying to cope with adolescence as best they could while my limited parenting capacity to deal with the emotional struggles teenagers have was compromised even further by financial difficulties. There is an undercurrent of panic in all of us. Now Erica is depending on me too.

The goalposts have changed. I spent the last twelve months fighting for my survival, praying that I would be around for my children for just a few more years. I wanted to live until Lisa was eighteen – as if eighteen would make a difference! There can never be a right time for a mother to leave her children. Now I am praying twice as hard for another eighteen years to be here for Erica.

I made the effort to get up early on Christmas morning to see my daughter and granddaughter open presents. In Fiona's face I saw her sadness – a distraught, pain-filled face reflected in my eyes. She was losing her family – no, she had *lost* her family.

Her boyfriend left, and when he did he took the only way Erica could stay in the home with her mum. Fiona needed him to be two parents in one and a loving partner, but it was too much for him and he left. My poor daughter was heartbroken.

I have to get better and quickly. I have major decisions to make, and I have to be fit to take on the next challenge in my life.

New Year, New Beginnings and New Ways of Thinking

On 14 January 2008, it was a very wintery, cold outside and freezing inside. Fiona handed Erica to me and asked me to care for her. She said she could not cope any more. I had seen this moment coming and had no doubts about the decision I was going to make – none whatsoever. There was never any other choice in my head. I wish I could promise to be there for Erica for ever, but I can only offer to love my granddaughter and provide stability for the rest of my life. I have done this before – I loved and provided for my own children. I just have to start again, that's all. I may be older and wiser, with more patience, but I have less stamina. But there is never a question of love. I have so much love for both my own daughter and Erica Lisa Angel.

9 February 2008

Two weeks ago mummy let you go;
She gave her gift to me.
She tried so hard to care for you;
But it wasn't meant to be.
Please, Erica, never blame your mum –
It's not her fault, you see.
Mummy is trapped in a world that only she can own.
And there she lives alone.
Mummy was brave to face the world and say,
"I cannot cope or care for you the way a Mummy should."
As she reached out for the very last time
She tried with all her heart,
But she couldn't quite touch you, little girl,
And with the hurt she fell apart.

Inside I too am falling apart. I know I have to accept all the help that is offered to me as I am still recovering from my treatment. My stamina is limited. I have lost the ability to protect Fiona as she has withdrawn from us all – a totally normal reaction to her partner leaving, and losing her child.

Fiona was unemployed and filled with sadness, she

decided a change of scenery was what she needed. She hoped London would bring wealth, fame, overnight success and happiness, so she headed for the big city. It is a familiar story. Years ago Adrian, my brother, headed off to the big city to then travel to Egypt to find the magic and mystery of the Pyramids. Thank goodness Mum reported him missing! We ended up being called to a London hospital. He was only thirteen at the time, and the *Birmingham Evening Mail* (newspaper) had read, 'Come Home, Bill Bailey' – (Adrian William Bailey) – front-page news.

Fiona felt there was nothing to keep her in the Midlands. The only people who can reach her are on the wrong side of the law, and she is vulnerable with a capital 'V'. Fiona had gone to London to find fame and work. She looked on the Internet for cheap room rentals, then she went with little money and ended up in a bathroom with a psychopath on the other side of the door. I only had time and enough credit to tell her to ring the police. I was lying in bed, two hours away, with Erica next to me; I was alone in the house and had no credit on my phone. I was mortified.

The next call I had was from the police: they had taken her to the station for her own safety, and they told me she was very naive and vulnerable. I was helpless and frightened for my child, as any parent would be. I learnt that having credit on the phone was an essential, like a gas bill – not for pointless texts, but for my own peace of mind. What if I had needed to call a doctor for Erica! As for Fiona, it was the start of many scrapes and near misses and many worries.

Luckily Lisa and I had some money between us when Erica had a reaction to ibuprofen and we needed to get her to the hospital. We had barely the taxi fare, but ever since then we have always kept a small stash of money in case of an emergency, though it is sometimes very difficult when you have a stash of money not to break into it.

Fiona's eyes are glazed most of the time, and sometimes I wanted so much for her to feel some maternal instinct for Erica, but her input to Erica's care always ends up on her terms and our relationship is under great strain. There is no doubt that Fiona loves Erica. Maternal instinct is an overpowering emotion. I am feeling frustrated and I think I have been in denial that my daughter's condition worsened by mental health issues has cut her off from me, her child and the rest of the family. When she was a child I had some influence over her decisions and I was able to protect her and keep her safe, but now as an adult I have no control at all over her safety. I could be her carer, in a sense, but only when she would let me. I thank God I am her first call whenever she is in trouble.

Fiona has been getting more vocal and aggressive towards me, and I now have to protect Erica from exposure to this. Sometimes this has meant I have had to compromise my loyalty to Fiona, but, as the world knows, the well-being of a child is paramount.

Fiona is fighting against emotions that she feels momentarily, but they never stay with her for long enough to change anything. The saddest part for me is seeing my child have some insight, but not enough to enable her to change anything. That is why Erica is with me. Fiona cannot feel outside her own body and mind at the moment and the person who loses out most is Fiona. Luckily my maternal instinct is and will always be to protect and care for my own daughter, whom I will love unconditionally for ever.

Money, Money, No Money, 18 February 2008

NO GAS, NO ELECTRIC, NO MONEY! I have decided to give up work, so I will have no forthcoming income. Are we sad? Are we poor? NO, because there's no such word as can't, as my mum always used to say. We haven't got heating, but we have clothes and blankets and cuddles; we haven't got light, but daytime is here. I spent wisely the last time we had money, and have healthy food in the cupboard. We have the park, the ducks, the world for free. The house is not cold, because it is full of love and laughter and singing. Today we struggle on and tomorrow is another day, another hoped-for dollar.

I made a big decision based on the stamina issue, and I knew this would be a risk, but I had no choice. I had to give up my career for now. My health, my family and my commitment to parenting a fourteen-month-old baby took over all my priorities. I needed all my energy and time to devote to these things and to ensure Erica was protected as much as possible from the emotional turmoil of separation from her mum. I was poor, but managing to keep my two teenagers, just about. It was difficult for the children to understand at times, especially when we sat freezing cold with no gas and a broken boiler.

Lisa had had to come home from her vocational dance school in Hertfordshire. She had to leave her friends and her boarding-school way of life. It was like St Trinian's at times, I think. Although I had no doubts about the fact I wanted Lisa to come back to reality and family values, it didn't help that she came back to a mum who was selling her jewellery for food. Luxuries were a thing of the past. Lisa's private education and her dance career seemed a dream away, and we woke up to yet another challenge that was to change all our lives for ever.

The manager in the NHS was doing everything she could to support my return to work, but I had made my decision. I had to save up all my emotional stamina for my own family. I wasn't prepared to compromise my registration as a nurse or let my family down. Nursing as a career is still about giving 110% and more; there is no room for any less at any time. The NMC (Nursing Midwifery Council) code of conduct (the nurse's bible) says a nurse takes responsibility for her own actions at all times and is accountable. I knew I had to leave work for now, and at that time, within my heavy heart, I thought it would be for ever.

Ali and Lisa were torn beyond belief. They believed that I was the wicked grandmother who had taken their sister's child off her. They were fighting her corner and still had faith in her. It was hard for them to accept that their sister was so unwell and so unhappy. They didn't know which way to turn, and sibling rivalry was confusing them even more. This was understandable as the focus was now on Erica and I had given up work to live on love. This was the period when the three of us and Erica seemed to have been catapulted into the ridiculous – but was it ridiculous? The lessons we all learnt at this time are invaluable and it was character-building for all of us. It forced us to face issues around the value of money, independence, motivation to work and self-respect.

The 'ridiculous' became in a lot of ways the sublime, and we learnt that fun is free if you spend happiness wisely.

I have juggled money and borrowed money, always worked and earned my own money, spent money and given it away. I have never saved for a rainy day, and so the rainy days to me were like raging thunderstorms. I comfort myself that after fifty years (half a century!) I am not a failure at managing money, but a success. Perhaps this isn't true in the conventional sense, but when I look back on what I have achieved I can see that I always got there in the end. Mine is not a story of inheritance or winning the lottery. (At one stage I was the only person who didn't belong to the works lottery syndicate, until the manager said I would be the only person left in the building to hold the fort if they won. He frightened me enough to make me think I ought to join the syndicate just in case.) But with drive, determination and some risk-taking, I have faced many financial challenges and come through smiling. Of course sometimes tears of frustration would cloud the sunny days. I have been exposed to ridicule, degradation and humiliation, but I am lucky that within my soul a small flame kept flickering, lighting the fire to help me fight for what I believe in, sustained by the core values that I was given as a child. I was determined to succeed, and my reward for working hard and studying for my nursing qualification was that I enjoyed my chosen career for thirty-three years.

What I have is happy memories, and nursing provided me with financial security. A comfortable lifestyle is all I ever wanted.

In my books there is always a message to readers, and this book is no exception. I hope to stimulate thought about how we perceive wealth. How do we treat and speak to people less fortunate than ourselves? How do we perceive status, or class? What is it actually like living on benefits? How do we define being poor? My definition of being poor is 'loneliness and isolation'. Without my family and friends I am the poorest person on earth.

In 2007 I couldn't afford to go to a salsa weekend in Blackpool and celebrate being well again. The last time I was in Blackpool I had had one dose of my chemotherapy.

My sadness did not last long. My friend Roz had started her own business selling salsa dancing shoes, and she had a proposition to make. Roz asked me to go to Blackpool with her and sell her shoes in the day; then I could salsa the night away and she would pay my board. I almost snapped her hand off in my excitement.

We had a very prosperous weekend. I absolutely loved fitting and advising ladies and men about the best salsa shoe for them. They were beautiful sparkly shoes – it was like the Cinderella story in real life. I made one mistake that did cause some hilarity: I sold two left shoes to a gentleman, but when he came back we exchanged them with a laugh and a giggle. There is always a funny story! I promised him I didn't think he had two left feet!

I had to work for my weekend, but I so enjoyed it and I was able to be with my wonderful salsa community.

Stuey Wuey and Lynney Wynney

I was in my financial swamp and Stuart and Lynn threw me a rope. Stuart worked away all week and needed a cleaner to get the house in order for the weekend every Friday. Lynn would pick me up and take me there. That cash was a lifeline in my time of need. They are good friends, never ever forgotten. Lynn remains a wonderful friend and we talk on a daily basis – always there for each other.

I married on 8 October 2010, and one of my dearest friends, Stuart, was taken from us on 8 October 2012 at the age of forty-four. He was a good man and a good friend, and I will never forget him. May he RIP – xxxxx.

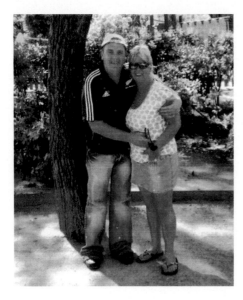

Stuey Wuey and Lynney Wynney, whom Lisa and I met up with in Barcelona in 2007 – such wonderful friends.

My Soulmate

My childhood from the age of eleven also changed drastically, emotionally and financially. My granddad had paid for me to go to a private school in my primary years, but the sudden change in the family when two parents became one stopped Mum's dreams and aspirations in their tracks. Dad had schizophrenia and he couldn't work. The private school gave me the discipline to work hard to survive when I moved to a secondary modern school. I loved my secondary school, and it was here I met my best friend, Janine, aged eleven.

Thirty-four years later to ease my financial problems Janine and Ian helped me to get a cheaper flat during my chemotherapy. We have always remained best friends, and I am godmother (or, as the girls call me, 'rock mother') to all her children. If you can have more than one soulmate, then Janine would be one of mine. In fact, Janine comes nearest to my definition of the one and only soulmate. Janine remembers the times when Dad would go off for walks in the middle of the night, and she remembers us both looking after Adrian, my brother, and Helen, my sister, in the school holidays. We went on holiday with both my mum and her parents, and we both had brothers named Adrian who were lost in tragic circumstances. You can't buy love and you can't buy happiness. I am rich, as I have a good and lasting friendship with Janine, and of course her husband, Ian.

These are just a few examples of their kindness, and so many other friends helped me too. I will never forget them – they know who they are.

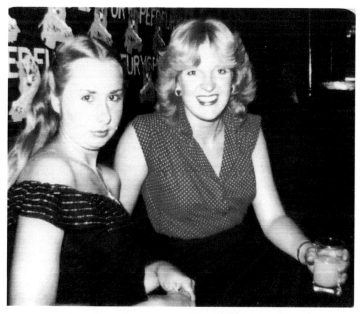

Janine and me on our Thursday night out at a nightclub in Birmingham in the 1970s.

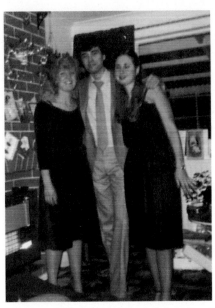

Me with Janine and her brother Adrian in the 1970s. In 1982 he was killed in a car accident aged twenty-one. Five days after Janine and Ian's wedding, we had to call them back off their honeymoon.

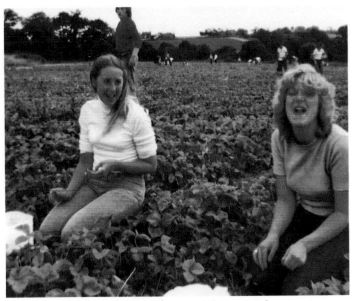

Janine and I strawberry picking in the 1970s.

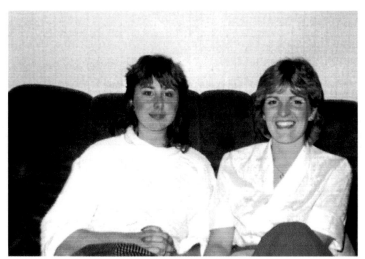

*Newly-weds in the 1980s, looking very married
and serious – ha ha.*

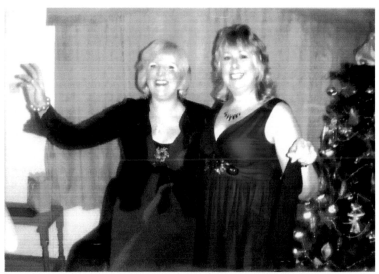

The celebration of half a century, December 2009.

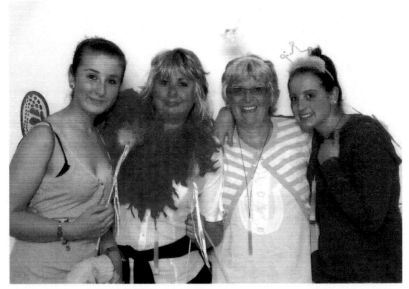

Me, Janine and our youngest daughters, Emily and Lisa, 2009. The Solstice Walk raising money for our local hospice.

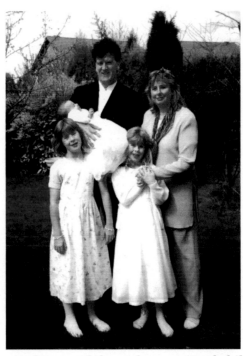

Janine and Ian and the girls – my 'Rockchildren'.

The Recipe of Life

Do we appreciate how much we have when we have the luxury of a healthy mind and body? Wouldn't it be great if all we had to worry about is 'Does my bum look big in this?'

When we are born we enter the world totally reliant on reflexes. We cry to communicate, and we are given cuteness to appeal to our birth mother and father so that they will pick our tiny defenceless bodies up and hold us close to them to make us feel safe. They hold us close to their hearts so that we can feel for the first time the heartbeat of someone who loves us, and then they feed us to sustain our existence. I really don't know if any parent can fully comprehend the responsibility that lies ahead.

As we proceed along life's path, our destiny evolves and for roughly eighteen years of our lives, perhaps more, perhaps less, our parents are often the most important people in our lives. However, a powerful influence lies ahead: opportunity. On paper it doesn't have the impact that a word like supercalifragilisticexpialidocious does, but *opportunity* does shape our lives. So we look into the eyes of that person who looks down at us with our future reflected in their eyes, and we say, "Where are you taking me? What path are you preparing for me?" And what opportunities have you planned for me? Genetics, birth experience, family function or dysfunction, education, opportunity, family values and our parents' expectations are the ingredients to just about complete the recipe of life. And a sprinkle of money would help. How much we get out of life's mixture depends on how much the opportunity ingredient makes the cake rise. And an extra drop of opportunity does make life taste a little better.

Opportunity requires money. In some Third World countries even the opportunity to live depends on donations of money, to help provide clean water, or vaccines to protect children against disease. I have always had the insight to know how much worse off others are. I say this to ensure there is not a whining element behind my story when I am describing my own period of financial hardship.

For a while my life revolved around payment cards. No way would I pay by direct debit. I had no control over my money, so bills got paid on the dot – but on my dot.

Every week I paid gas, electric, water and TV-licence instalments, but my rent and community tax were now taken into account with my benefits. Child tax credit and child benefit helped me to keep my head above water, and I could live. I had a television, and I couldn't help but notice that every advertisement is aimed at people with a disposable income. I felt for parents at Christmas confronted by advertisements for expensive toys. 'Minimalistic' to me was not a design idea; for me and many others it was a necessity.

I had flown to Cancer Planet and now I was in my rocket to Planet Minimalist. It was a challenge and at times it meant isolation. I don't drink or smoke, so a night out was sometimes achievable – tap water is free in a pub.

I am one of the lucky ones, yet again because of my mum – perhaps I should say because of positive parenting, which includes Dad too.

Mum gave me as a child the strength to fight adversity in any form. How she did this was very simple. She showed me by being the strong positive woman she is – and she has been through her own adversity. As a mum she never criticised me or teased me or threatened me; she praised me and she believed in me. She never believed in 'can't'. Mum had strict guidelines and boundaries and these were based on good principles. My manners – treating people with respect – have stood me in good stead in my life. I will always remember stopping off at a café when we were going on holiday and Adrian burped – ha! ha! We were immediately ushered out to the car – no drink, no food – and Adrian had a right flea in his ear.

Mum fought to give us opportunities; she maintained our beautiful home and went without luxuries so we could live in comfort; she saved all year so we could have one fun holiday and an enjoyable Christmas. We had it all: we had a happy childhood, and we knew we were loved because every day she told us so.

"All the money in the world couldn't buy my Sharon."

"All the money in the world couldn't buy my Helen."

"All the money in the world couldn't buy my Adrian."

And now Helen and I say it to our own children because its TRUE.

One of the most crucial ingredients of our early years and childhood is the experience of positive, loving parenting. This sets the course for how we move from childhood to adulthood.

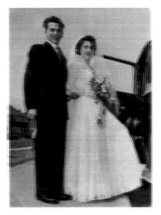

Meet the parents.
Mum and Dad, happy on their
wedding day.
If Mum had a crystal ball,
maybe her smile would not
have been so bright.

DEAR PARENT

What are your plans for me?
I am your child, you see.
I cannot live without you,
Your love and stability.

Whatever our family tree describes –
One person, two or three –
I need your hugs when I am sad.
One special person just for me!

Please take me places for me to play,
Meet new friends and learn to share.
One special gift that you can give me
Is the ability to care.

Send me to school and teach me at home;
Show me what you can do.
I am totally reliant on your praise and guidance –
All I want is to be like you.

The time has come: I am ready to fly.
Wish me luck in life as you wave goodbye.
Please don't turn away, Mum. I will always need you there.
No one can replace our special bond that we will always share.

My Mum

I saw my mum fight to keep what she had worked for. Her own father had his own business, and Mum worked hard every day for every penny she was paid, handling large bales of hessian. Life was hard, especially after 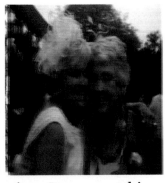 Dad left us at the age of thirty-nine. It was not his choice to leave us, but life's fateful events took him from us. His unfair destiny was mental illness. We did suffer from the loss of our father. He was lost in mind, even when he was there in body – a helpless, dependent father. That experience possibly had some effect on my future failed relationships.

Mum had our best interest at heart always, and we were not spoiled – only spoiled with love. Mum made sure Christmases were the same for us as for everybody else in the street, with turkey dinners, presents in our stockings, and fun and laughter. We had a holiday every year in a caravan, with a pound a day to spend on ice cream and a drink in the club at night. Benny from *Crossroads* used to go to the same caravan site as we did. We used to make loads of sandwiches and, take them to the beach, and I would be the one to carry the bloomin' dinghy! We had enough money for one ice cream a day; and Mum made us brave the rain and took us on the beach until the sun shone again, because we didn't have spare money to waste on a rainy day in arcades.

We always celebrated our birthdays in style. Mum would pile all our friends in the car (this was before seat belts) and take us to the park. We had the traditional blancmange, jellies and ice cream.

We had cherryade in wine glasses on a Sunday from the milkman, and chocolate cake and custard from the bread man. This was our big treat.

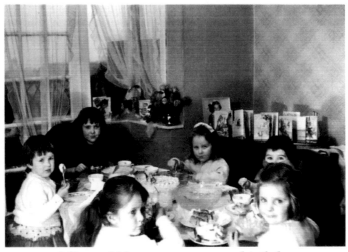

Jelly and blancmange on my birthday.

I remember Mum hiding in the lobby (what we called our cloakroom) because she couldn't afford to pay the insurance man, but when my sister Helen opened the door the caller was a neighbour. Then Helen opened the lobby door and standing there in the dark was Mum. Ha ha! We laugh now. And I remember the time when Mum had 75 pence for a joint of meat, and the butcher weighed every pork joint in the shop because it had to be dead on 75 pence and no more.

We sometimes had to put Fine Fare shopping bags over Adrian's terry-towelling nappies. Helen told me he used to wear her nighties – oh, dearie me!

Helen also remembers Dad losing his temper with Mum and throwing a dinner over her and shouting at Adrian. I am glad she cannot remember everything else, but I can. I remember wondering what was happening as doors were smashed and things were being thrown out of the window. Mum cried a lot, and Dad was very often in bed, just lying there dirty. I would stand at the bedroom door looking at the man in the bed and feel guilty because I hated my own father.

Eventually Dad was sectioned under the Mental Health Act. In a sad way it was a relief at last not to be in such an unpredictable environment any more.

Childhood experiences do influence the way you live your adulthood life. So much depends on the messages parents give their children. Through no fault of his, Dad was a dependant; his ability to be a role model came to an end when mental illness changed this eccentric, gentle, loving man into a man taken over by paranoia, anger, violence and madness. My dad was diagnosed with paranoid schizophrenia.

DAD

The disease of the mind is hard to define
An island separated
By an ocean in turmoil
That stops your mind meeting mine
In the early days we swam in a calm clear blue sea
My sister, my brother, and me
We would swim to the shore and rest on the softest sand
A family together united hand in hand
But one cold and thunderous volatile grey day
The ocean became angry and swept the family away
A wild and destructive wave came sweeping over me
A family all drowning in sadness and unpredictability
In your final years and your final days
The sea became calm we swam through the waves
To rest on the shore on the soft, soft sand
At last we could reach you united again we stand
I turn to my sister as a bright light begins to shine
I say to her
I have waited
It has taken a lifetime
But I just captured a moment
A moment so sublime
It was that precious moment when
At last
Dad's mind meets mine
Meets mine.

I saw my mum devastated and crying with frustration. When Dad was sectioned to a psychiatric hospital Mum became Mum and Dad. She became stronger, parenting as best she could. Dad was still in our lives as Mum remained loyal to him. This experience influenced my earliest adult experiences in relationships. I developed the strength from my mum to survive and become self-sufficient, able to manage no matter what the situation I was in, whether married, divorced, single, not single, healthy or dealing with cancer. From Dad – I recognised love as need rather than love. I have spent my life struggling with relationships and that's another story.

Adrian (my brother) had only us women to adore him. He was a cute little baby and an adorable funny little boy, and he made us laugh through all the sad, bad times. He inherited Dad's musical talent and his illness. Music has been a massive influence in all our lives.

In his younger years Adrian, my brother, sang as frontman in a Beatles-type line-up. As manager of the group, I used to get the band gigs raising money for local charities. They did get their three minutes of fame on *Daytime Live*, 'singing out' the programme with a classic Beatles song: 'A Hard Day's Night'. Lulu and Sandie Shaw were the other guests. It was all very exciting. We keep replaying that video now to remember my beautiful brother. He wasn't sectioned under the Mental Health Act, but at thirty-nine years of age, on 26 February 2009, he took his own life. He had started hearing voices and was not prepared to repeat history and live with schizophrenia like his own dad, and love was to deal him a bitter blow too.

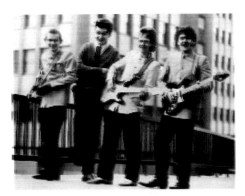

The Diversions, about 1981.

A year earlier to the day Adrian took his own life; he was helping me start my new life. On 26 February 2008 I moved into a council property. It is an ideal house in a quiet village. Many of the villagers have lived there all their lives. There is a local shop, a Tesco Express, a saddler, a Chinese takeaway and a chip shop in walking distance. There is a park, and a mother-and-toddler group at the village church.

Adrian and I decorated one bedroom in a day; me and the children all slept in the one room. The rest of the upstairs needed tender loving care and quickly. As Adrian filled holes in the walls, I followed him around with a paintbrush. At one point I looked around to find Mum balancing on the side of the bath, stripping old wallpaper. Mike (my stepdad) pottered for weeks ahead, fixing plugs and shelves and doors. I think he enjoyed the solitary peace. He helped me such a lot in those first few months, and I needed that help.

I was so proud of my new home. If it moved, I painted it – even the outside of the house and the wall at the end of the garden! I made my own rockery and painted the rocks white too. Erica would go to her granddad's, and as soon as she went the paint pot was out. I decorated the hall, stairs and landing in magnificent magnolia. The reward as I saw the house grow into a home was a wonderful feeling. Ali slept in the front downstairs room, but at this time we had no carpets, only wooden floors and tiling. I painted the wooden floor white in the bathroom – it was quite effective really, very nautical. I had the bare essentials, and we had a very small TV, fridge, microwave and washing machine.

Home Start not only supported with advice about handling my debts (and, of course, the creditors), but carpeted my bedroom and Lisa's bedroom, and a few months' later arranged for Erica and me to go on a subsidised Home Start holiday at a Haven site for a break in a caravan. We lived on £80 for the week (just over £10 a day) for food, nappies, drinks and bus fares. We brought pebbles home from the beach to give as presents.

During my cancer treatment I had met a very old friend in a famous store at the till – Diane. I used to frequent the coffee shop in this store after a chemo session for a very special treat: a yummy latte, one of the only tasty things I could stand and digest. Di and I had both worked as midwives together; also we were both of us in labour on the same day – I was having Fiona, and Di was having double trouble twin girls. Di was now working with the Carers Association and, because of my caring role for Fiona and Erica, she referred me to a colleague for a carer's assessment.

My key worker was so resourceful and supported an application to particular trusts that support nurses in times of hardship, and so I managed to purchase a cooker and a sofa and other household commodities.

I was also invited to the Carers Association support groups, and I enjoyed my time there when Erica was at nursery. I also gave talks to groups in the area about becoming an author. I really enjoyed sharing my ability to 'write from the heart'. Another social opportunity for the next two years was provided by the children's centre, and I think it saved my sanity. On family day, parents and children went to play during the morning with their baby or toddler, and we formed friendships, talked and supported each other. Then we had lunch. Family day was a great idea. Most importantly there was comradeship instead of what could have been isolation from the world. I will always remember the happy welcoming faces of the people I met there and how they made a big impact on my life and Erica's.

It might have been there that my creativity first came to the forefront, as I attempted to make robots and paint pictures. I even joined in the adult-learning course on scrapbook-making. I hasten to add that, even though the excitement and enthusiasm was there to reach out to my hidden talents, I was reassured that the career path I had taken up to now was the right one: I was still pretty useless at making things. But in the back of my mind I was thinking, 'I wish I could actually publish my journal.' I wondered, 'Could I?'

I was no longer working (my official date of finishing work was the end of January 2008). I never thought I would work again, and it was at this time I began to have cognitive behaviour therapy. I had asked for professional help, counselling, but talking again about my past was not the answer. I hadn't time now to go back over old ground. I had worked out what had influenced my failed relationships, and I had faced up to the cancer and written all my experiences down on paper. Actually I was comfortable in my victim mode. It meant I could hibernate from the world and feel sorry for myself, but there was a catch: I had to shape up emotionally because I had Erica to raise into a healthy child. Her emotional health was just as important as her physical health, and I knew that her childhood experiences would affect her adult life. I wanted her to have memories of a happy nan, smiling and making the best of life, enjoying the simple things as well as always striving for better things. I wanted Erica to venture into life with the confidence to try and never give up, just as I had seen my own mum do. She never gave up on her dreams, on us or on herself. She was a strong influence in my life.

My own children had seen my determination and strength of character in the pre-cancer times of their childhood when stamina was not an issue. Youth had been on my side and I had the desire to give my own children chances. If they excelled at something, I would support them all the way. I wanted them to enjoy every waking day, and I wanted them to enjoy earning their money, loving going to work, just as I did.

When I was at the bus stop on my way to my first appointment I just stood there thinking, 'I don't want to get better.' I felt safe in a victim bubble of sadness. Nobody expected anything from me. I wanted to bow my head and walk past life. I only needed the sanctuary of my new home, Erica, my children and the rest of my family.

I turned up to that appointment with food down my top, odd socks on my feet (although that was nothing new in my house), and no make-up. I had no energy to drag myself out of the hole – only enough to look after Erica. But I did go to the appointment. I knew that appointments for mental-health services were like gold dust. The staff were under enormous pressure and I respected my fellow colleagues, so I turned up, and each week I did the tasks I was set, and gradually I realised where I had been and where I was going, and eventually I could see the pot of gold at the end of the rainbow. That was the Sharon Rose I knew – the Sharon Rose my family and friends knew and loved.

I scrubbed up, I learnt to problem-solve, and, most importantly of all, I started to set myself some goals.

Mick Cope, author of *Coaching to Success* (2010), suggests your goals should be (1) subjective, about you; (2) singular, one thing at a time; (3) small, achievable and manageable; (4) specific, measurable; and (5) significant, likely to have an impact on you.

I love the bag-of-sweets scenario. The simple task of not buying a packet of sweets from the shop one morning may not seem important, but it might have a profound impact on somebody's life. Not buying the sweets that day meant they could say no. Therefore they could say no the next day too, and the day after that, and for 100 days, and a new habit might be formed: buying an apple instead of sweets. This would mean a lower calorific intake, leading to weight loss, better health, and perhaps a longer, more useful life.

The moral of the story is 'No matter how small the goal, it can have a major impact on improving your own life.'

Life is fragile, so handle with care! Plan short-term, realistic but challenging goals. I realised a lack of goals had led to feelings of depression. I needed goals to motivate me and provide me with a sense of meaning, and to boost my confidence as and when I achieved them.

I can't say having Erica came anywhere in the negative, because Erica was an angel who shone the light into my future.

Pride and Prejudice

It hurt sometimes to have no money in my pocket. I was confined to how far I could walk as I had no transport and the bus fare into town was £3.60 return. This could pay for at least two days' shopping. Unless the journey was essential I wouldn't travel, but then of course the loneliness and isolation became more intensified. I had sold all my jewellery to pay for food and I had gas and electric meters installed because direct debits were a liability if the money wasn't in the bank to pay the bills. At one time I had extra-ridiculous bank charges amounting to enough to pay for a month's shopping. The benefits system does its job: it helps you live just below the poverty line, no more, no less. And existence on benefits is outside the bubble that working folk live in. No, I couldn't meet for coffee; no, I couldn't meet for lunch – not any more. Window-shopping was the norm, and I strolled around charity shops looking for Christmas presents. That year Erica had a doll's house and furniture, and many other second-hand toys brought her much joy and pleasure for a minimal price.

You do not realise what being a minority means until you are in the minority. The majority of people struggle at some time in their life financially, but even the lives of affluent people are centred too much around wealth. Wherever we look we are being encouraged to spend money, and there are the heartless moneylenders that jump on the bandwagon and set up high-interest loans to enable people to feel that at least they are part of the twenty-first century. The poor and wealthy are divided, and some of the super-wealthy are on a different planet altogether.

Shopping became easier as I used to visit the 'mummy shop' and had exactly £25 to spend – the minimum amount for delivery. Every time I went shopping I tried to add up the amount in my head, but I should have taken a calculator because I often had to walk back around putting food items back on the shelves. On one occasion I had more than £25 so I didn't have to do the routine trip back around the shop – I didn't know whether to laugh or cry, especially when the sales assistant actually commented on the fact that I didn't have to take any items back.

I remember as clear as day a time when I cried openly, sitting on a bus amongst familiar faces my bus buddies. The other passengers remained silent, and my tears were the only sound. Some people looked away, and some looked at me aghast at the emotional outburst as I fought for my dignity. I had queued that day and the bus was crowded with people returning home after work. I had searched for the bus fare home and gave the driver £1.80 in small change. There was a look of disgust in the driver's eyes, and he shouted at me, telling me I was stupid to bring this change at his busiest time. I couldn't see anything through tears, and a women behind me rescued me and consoled me and gave the driver 50 pence. I remember defending myself, repeating how I used to be a nurse and worked hard, but the driver saw someone who was giving up, not bothered about herself, unkempt, who had dinner down her top, and he treated me like something he had wiped off his shoe. I saw judgemental bigotry, and I swore I would never make anyone less fortunate than myself feel as I did that day. I felt humiliated. What was I coming to? This was a turning point for me.

Single Salsa Survivor

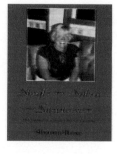

The book *Single Salsa Survivor: The Journal of a Breast Cancer Survivor* was published in 2010.

My community psychiatric nurse asked me what I would like to achieve post-cancer and during remission. I said I wanted to try to see if my book was worth publishing. My aim was to give women strength to cope with a diagnosis of breast cancer and get through the treatment and, when it is all over, hope for their future. As I became stronger in body and soul I saw an advert from a publisher in the magazine *Candis*. The advert invited authors to send their manuscript in and they would see if they could publish the book. I did just that, and the rest is now history thanks to Arthur H. Stockwell Ltd.

I couldn't believe it when the letter came back and said yes. I was so excited about the prospect of seeing my book on the shelves in our leading book stores, and my intention was to reach as many women as possible who may benefit from reading the book. My self-esteem began to grow; life was settling down. I had a supportive man friend in my life, and Erica and I were adapting to what was now a mother–daughter relationship. I now had three daughters, in a sense, and I loved them all the same.

I was making decisions again, looking forward. I was feeling better mentally and emotionally. I had learnt that life cannot stand still in a static time zone for ever. My short-term goal (and my long-term goal) was to stay alive, but I couldn't survive daily living without some new short-term goals to challenge me, to inspire a spark of life in me. No goals meant no moving on from grief, and grief is a big part of the process of surviving cancer and what I call the 'loss of my mortality'.

The book was due out on 31 March. I had decided from the start that 20% of my royalties would go to Cancer Research UK. It is the largest cancer charity in the UK, and without their expertise and research into cancer prevention and treatment I would not be one of the survivors.

I hadn't been working, but now I needed something to stimulate my own brain back into action. I wanted something that I enjoyed doing – something close to my heart – so I began writing my second book, telling the story of my relationship with a widower, Chris, whose wife had lost her battle against breast cancer. Their daughter Faith had escaped her own grief by taking photos of beauty in the garden and editing them. These photos of flowers are magical. Faith had taken to photography as I had taken to creative writing, her photos and my words reflecting our depth of feelings. We produced beautiful meaningful bookmarks for charity, but I never made a penny for myself. I have never been great at selling even a raffle ticket – but, oh, I did gain so much pleasure in this year through raising money for national and local cancer charities.

I also offered to do a creative-writing session at the carers' group, and this was so rewarding to me and those taking part. This was when the bookmarks came into their own. I talked about my book and the subject area of remission in cancer, and the importance of positive thoughts and positive emotions in helping people through the difficult situations and challenges life brings. I then worked with the group and asked them not to think about being an author or expert in the English language, but to write from the heart as I have done. I had bookmarks made with the caption 'I CARE FOR YOU' and the group wrote about their positive emotions regarding the person they cared for. I had so much back from these sessions, and some of the poetry written by the people who attended them was heart-moving. Any one of us can express our feelings in the written word if we just listen to our hearts.

"Write your thoughts down straight away
Before your dreams are yesterday."

April 2010

Chris moved in and I claimed my NHS pension.

I paid off my creditors and, for the first time in about thirty years, I owed no one any money. My life had turned around full circle. I returned to work as a working mum again, and I had aspirations for the future.

I had learnt very hard lessons about surviving on the last food product in the cupboard and the last penny in my purse. I had learnt not to look at things I couldn't afford. I had made the very best of fun out of things that cost nothing, such as a walk in the park or spending quality time with friends. My mum and stepdad's caravan in Wales again came in for some good use, and Erica had the chance to build sandcastles, jump over the waves and join in the children's disco in the caravan-site clubhouse. Our drinks cost only 30 pence – a blackcurrant and soda for me and a fruit shot for Erica – and we were happy.

My life is my inspiration to succeed – my family, my children, my granddaughter, my long-term career in the NHS, my relationships (the good, the bad and the ugly), music, dancing (especially salsa), my journey through stages of breast cancer and remission, and, of course, my own favourite iconic authors.

On holiday I took Richard Branson with me. I used to say to Chris, Richard Branson says this and that, and Chris used to say, "Don't bring that man on holiday again!" I tried to get some tips from the man himself from his book *Screw It, Lets Do It*, and I would be sitting on the beach looking out to sea and then quote from Richard Branson's book and tell Chris I felt a great affinity with his business sense. Chris listened attentively, as any good partner would, but we couldn't understand how Richard Branson was so rich and I was not and we would laugh together.

RICHARD BRANSON'S ETHOS

Change the world, even in a small way.
Make a difference and help others.
Do no harm.
Always think what you can do to help.

Richard Branson also quoted the following in his book, "*Screw It, Let's Do It*":

'Just do it.'
'Think yes, not no.'
'Have goals.'
'Stand on your own two feet.'
'Be loyal.'
'Live life to the full.'
'Nothing ventured, nothing gained.'
'Use a notebook.'

So Richard is of my way of thinking. He carried his notebook around with him, I am sure, jotting down inspirational thoughts about how to run a successful eco-friendly business, and so he became an iconic, very wealthy businessman; and, simply, I haven't.

I have also been inspired by Susan Jeffers and her self-help books – particularly *"Feel the Fear and Do It Anyway"*. Pushing through fear, she says, is less frightening than living with the underlying fear that comes with helplessness. In this book there is a chapter about 'boxes'. I found the boxes an interesting concept, and explained the idea to my children. They laughed at me then, but years later have mentioned on numerous occasions the famous boxes. The theory is that if you fill your life totally with one and only one focus, then when you lose that one focus the loss is of greater significance and impact. But if you have a life full of many different boxes, each filled with one thing – for example, relationships, family, faith, career, children, hobbies, then when one box is lost the other boxes make the loss bearable and easier to cope with. You can still give each box 100% when you are within the realms of the box in question.

"Embracing Uncertainty", also by Susan Jeffers, discusses the word maybe. This very simple word can take away all expectations and make views on life so much more simple. I applied the theory to my experience of cancer: maybe I will survive cancer; maybe I won't. I do not know. But while I am living I can make my life count, giving 100% to everything I do. With that way of thinking, my life has improved 100%. Stay positive!

My third inspiration is the community psychiatric nurse who guided me through cognitive behaviour therapy, John – to you I thank you.

Ali, My Son

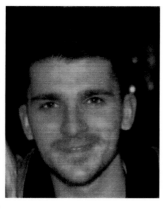

Ali rarely cried as a baby, played happily made friends easily, worked hard at school, scored 100 goals in one season and put up with his mum running up the pitch shouting, "Shoot, Ali, shoot!" Ali loved his home, his sisters, his mum, Wales (especially Porthmadog, or should I say Port Maggots?) and he loved his stepdad, Paul.

He was good at every sport, and if he had a bad day at golf he would say to me, "Mum, I've lost my swing.

He came to all Lisa's shows and dance festivals (he was bought up in the arts) and Lisa went to every football match. Then just when adolescence started to complicate his life, so did circumstance; and at the same time Ali lost his playmate to boarding school and his mate through marital separation. And his stepdad rejected him – the man he had looked up to since the age of ten months. Just when it seemed as though things couldn't get any worse, his mum got cancer – she lost that stamina that kept her running up the pitch and she cried at night when the world was asleep and only he could hear.

Ali was the only one who knew how ill I was. He was the only one who heard my sobs and saw my tears. He was the one left to see the fear in my eyes on a daily basis. He missed Lisa, but Fiona had moved back in and he loved her despite her sometimes random ways. We all loved her for her random ways and her leopard-skin knickers, and we all laughed together most of the time as she walked around in them without a care in the world.

On the positive side, Ali had a great fun teenage

time in our small apartment in town. Many times there were bodies asleep in every corner of our flat when I came home, and I loved it. I have never in my life met such lovely teenagers – harmless happy boys and girls that had a bond of friendship that I could see would never falter. I provided them with a safe haven where they could enjoy their youth in comfort and safety. Everybody thought I was crazy, but hearing them laugh and joke gave me all the pleasure in the world. When one of these beautiful boys was killed in a car accident, they congregated in my flat, all of them, to share their grief.

Ali had been unwell with depression, which is understandable when you look at the circumstances this teenager was in. His stamina had suffered, and this had affected his football skills. I saw his confidence fall. Once as he entered the box to score a goal he stopped right in front of my eyes. My son needed help. Luckily he had so many friends, and gradually he pulled through the worst.

When I wore dark glasses on a summer's day in August it wasn't to hide the glare of the sun; it was to hide the constant tears I shed as I drove my son to the college to change his career path. He wanted to be a fireman, but depression and antidepressants were on his medical records, so uniformed services were out of the question. Now as depression was affecting his CV I wanted him out of it. I wanted him not to see me crying any more.

When he said he wanted to work abroad, I said, "Son, that's the best idea yet. Go for it. Take a risk. The worst scenario is that you will have to come home after a few days in the sun."

This was in the summer of 2007, a year after my treatment for cancer. I had returned to work and was feeling very positive about life. I had an insurance policy that I cashed in, and I was able to buy Ali a friend's car for his eighteenth birthday. Although he hadn't passed his test it seemed like a good idea at the time. I had ordered a dining table and sofa with the rest of the money. I used the cancer excuse for my impulsiveness, but really I had always been impulsive – so what did I do? I cancelled the sofa, kept the dining table, and set off to Magaluf with Lisa and my friend Jill, who was in plaster up to her thigh due to a netball injury that put her salsa on hold for a while. It was Lisa's sixteenth-birthday treat, and I also wanted to see for myself that Ali was OK. Yes, I know: random.

Well, Jill couldn't face the week. We were in a hotel that was probably on the programme *Holidays from Hell* and was Fawlty Towers. Jill was restricted by her plaster of Paris, and she hated the place so she took the next plane home.

Lisa and I had the greatest mum-and-daughter holiday. We laughed and danced the night away, but the funniest time was when we turned up at Ali's apartment block. I knew the block but not the number, and we had to shout, "Ali!" on every floor until a head popped out of a door and said "Mum, what are you doing here?"

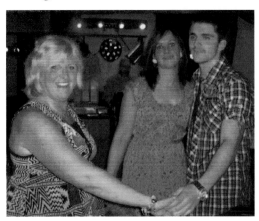

Me, Ali and Leanne at his twenty-first birthday party.

"I'm on holiday with your sister, son," I said. "We just happened to drop in."

He was enjoying life at last, and for a while escaping the misery of the last few months and years. When he came home he managed to get a job in a matter of days, and with his money he entered the world of responsibility. Without a question he paid his way.

What I didn't know then was that besides all that football he also had the dream to sing. Now we are going to his gigs. Nobody escapes the Bailey family musicality! I am lucky to have seen him grow into the man he is today. At twenty-one he owns his own house with his girlfriend, who is a nurse. They are engaged to be married, so I'd better start saving and getting the hat ready.

Five Years On, 2010

I married Chris, and we had a traditional-but-wacky

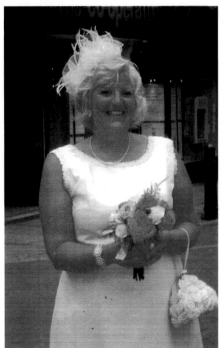

wedding day. I was happy and positive. My life had turned around. It was a moment of contentment.

It's a good thing I didn't have a crystal ball – my smile would never have been so bright.

Five years on I was sitting in my hairdresser's waiting to be transformed ready to catch a train to London with other cancer survivors in the UK to the launch of the Cancer Research UK Race for Life, 2011. I had been there in 2006 (as related in *Single Salsa Survivor*), dancing in the warm-up, surrounded by my friends, and racing to give me and other cancer sufferers the chance to experience the gift of life. In 2010 I got on stage and did a salsa warm-up for the thousands of runners and walkers that day. Cancer Research Race for Life, 2011 'Join the Girls'. During those five years, the scientists had been diligently working to cure cancer and to improve cancer treatment. For example, there are now shorter radiotherapy courses – the physical pain of radiotherapy is still the same, but fewer visits to the cancer centre mean there is less trauma and emotional pain.

At last, hair done, I was on the train, sitting opposite my youngest daughter, Lisa.

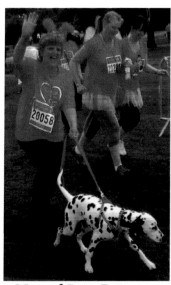

Me and Rose Button at the finishing line, 2011.

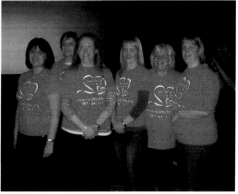

Race for Life, 2011, cancer survivors.

Lisa's Story

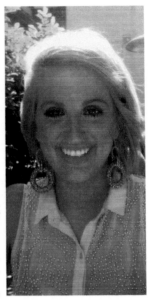

Lisa life has been extraordinary, and because of her extraordinary life mine has been extraordinary too. It all started when Lisa started ballet class (as did Fiona) at the age of four. Little did I know then that this tiny four-year-old was to blossom into a wonderful dancer and take me with her on the kind of journey you usually only read of in fairy tales.

I suppose the film *Billy Elliot* is a modern fairy tale. It showed how a working-class boy was able to follow his dream and become a successful dancer. Since then Simon Cowell has been the catalyst for talented performers to have their chance. Maybe it is not so important to have money and influential contacts as it once was.

I look out of the window and drift off to reflect on Lisa's story. I hope this part of the story creates debate and discussion. My choices in relation to Lisa's future have been made. It might have been better if I had done things differently, but, you know what, probably not. As I have said before, the Bailey family has the good fortune to be naturally musically talented, but the family also has a history of mental health problems. This time a little star was born – my star. As children we were bought up with *Singin' in the Rain* and *Hello Dolly*! We sang in the house; we sang in the car. We were so happy. But I never dreamt that my daughter would create such a charged atmosphere as she danced on the stage. When she danced to 'Papa Can You Hear Me?' by Barbra Streisand, the theatre would be silent, engulfed in the aura, mesmerised by her interpretation of the music through dance.

Lisa, at the age of seven, was accepted by the Royal Ballet School Junior Associates in Birmingham; and until she was thirteen we would be at football in the morning, Lisa would get dressed for ballet in the car, taking off muddy wellies and putting on her pretty pink leather ballet shoes, and she would dance for at least three hours solid without a murmur of pain or tiredness. She thrived on every opportunity to dance, and to see such commitment, loyalty and enthusiasm in such a young person convinced me that it was from deep within her soul, and I did everything to support her. The social side for me meant coffee and chats every Saturday in Birmingham coffee shops, with fellow proud mums and dads. Every August we would meet in Stratford-upon-Avon, one of my favourite places in the UK (another is Bournemouth). I made friendships there that lasted all those years. When we talked about sequins and pointe shoes and auditions it was my escapism from the norm. As a nurse I spent most of the week dealing with illness – a world so many miles apart from sequins and pirouettes. I loved that contrast. I loved the fact I didn't have a clue about dance, because it made me feel so much better if I knew nothing. I felt reassured that all this talent was not a result of the pushy-mum syndrome; it was totally Lisa's choice. But she couldn't get to auditions on her own, or dance festivals, so her dad and I had to make the decision to give her our commitment of time and moral support, and financially.

I had achieved my career aspirations, and when the three children were still very young I went to university for a year to study for my diploma in professional nursing, community health studies and health visiting. I was the main wage earner and bills had to be paid.

I had three children and never forgot that fact. All of them were encouraged in their own interest: Fiona and her singing competitions, Ali and his football, and

Lisa and her ballet. My life revolved around work and the children's extra-curricular activities. I was asked many times, "What do you do for yourself?" and my answer was always, "Exactly what I always wanted to do, and that is I take pride in bringing up my children the best I can to be happy healthy adults who will eventually have the confidence and the daily living skills to live without me."

I must admit it took me until the age of forty-five to find my passion for dancing salsa, and I never looked back.

I never saved for the future when I was well and cancer-free. I always lived for the now. When money became a worry Lisa's dad and I sold our house of six years and returned to the very same street we left six years before. We were now only a few doors away from our old house. Thank God we hadn't fallen out with the neighbours! They sent us off with a farewell committee and they welcomed us back six years later. That was funny really. Wherever I lay my hat, that's my home – even in the same street.

The money problem had come about for two reasons. One was the fact I had to see Lisa perform at every opportunity, and Lisa had been chosen to appear in *Still Life at the Penguin Café*, a ballet performed by Birmingham Royal Ballet, directed by David Bintley. Lisa was chosen to perform in London at Sadler's Wells, Sunderland and Plymouth, and then she returned for a gala performance and the reopening of the Birmingham Hippodrome. Lisa was the only child on the stage with principal ballerinas, and no mistake would have gone unnoticed. I wish I could see every performance again. She managed all the steps without a hitch. My heart was bursting with pride and awe. At the end of each performance Lisa took her memorable curtain call. I still cannot believe we had the opportunity to be part of this magic – and Lisa felt the same with all her heart.

Her reward was a Beanie. I would stand at the stage door clutching this present, waiting with pride. Such a simple reward with a powerful message.

Just a month later Lisa was chosen to play one of the children in the famous Christmas ballet *The Nutcracker*. During all fourteen performances I sat in the box or the circle or the stalls, and I never missed seeing my girl come on stage and celebrate Christmas every day. It was a little bit of a standing joke, I must admit: if someone had a spare ticket in the box for a matinee, I would jump up and say, "Yes, I will have it!" And then on the day the cast of children were in the wings and one of the children would say to Lisa, "Your mum's in the audience again."

I spent a lot of my hard-earned cash. We all went as a family, and the good seats at the ballet are not cheap.

So instead of worrying for years about money, we moved back to a street we knew – cheaper house and cheaper living – and loved and had no debts. Do I have any regrets? None at all.

As we get older, life gets a little harder. If dreams are to come true, it depends on the individual. Lisa was getting second auditions for White Lodge Royal Ballet School and Elmhurst School for Dance, Surrey, but I always remember the time one of the dance directors of the school told us the truth: ballerinas have to have the exact tools for the job. Loyalty, commitment and enthusiasm were not enough. Even good technique could no longer carry everything a dancer needs to be a ballerina. No, there is one final part of the success jigsaw, and that is physique. In those influential teenager years it is always a worry that determination to achieve the perfect ballerina's body can lead to disaster, with bulimia or anorexia. Lisa had something or other wrong with the measurements of her middle trunk area, so ballet scholarships were becoming a dream of the past. Lisa was offered places on all the musical-theatre dance courses that incorporated jazz dance. Ballet provides the basis for all other dance, and Lisa was an all-rounder.

It was for numerous reasons that I came to the next big decision of our family's lifetime. There were other private things that were brewing, and they influenced my decision.

I had seen my daughter focus totally on dance all her life. She had chosen her dance class over parties or days out. We never missed a class. Lisa learnt from her childhood never to give up on what you believe in. I was not prepared to give up for Lisa. My child was getting rejected for ballet scholarships and accepted for musical theatre and dance. It is a crazy system just to have scholarships for ballet! I took a risk, made a big decision, and in October 2004 drove down to Hertfordshire and left my third-born at boarding school. We had sold our house for Lisa. It was the last joint decision my husband and I made. Our marriage was over. There were no arguments about who had what or how much, because the last thing we both agreed on was both of us taking a risk and supporting our daughter for one year at vocational school.

A Little Tale of an Unexpected Legacy

Granddad Rose gave me elocution lessons in preparation for when I took over his business, but when I told him I wanted to be a nurse he was really cross with me. He wouldn't speak to me for a while, but he came round to the idea when Mum gave him a talking-to.

There is a story about how my Granddad Rose helped me in a very mysterious way twenty-two years after he died. He was my guardian angel when he was alive, and I was with him by his side when he died. My Granddad Rose never went on holiday he worked until he could no longer walk even with his Zimmer frame. He gave me my first Saturday job and I did get a telling-off when I sent all his faithful regular customers invoices to remind them they needed to pay us. That made me chuckle. He adored and loved me, and I knew it even if he was a bit grumpy. We loved each other. He gave me away on my first wedding because it felt right. He had been like a father to me, and Dad was really ill at the time as he wouldn't take his medication.

Granddad Rose had a great work ethic and he believed in the best. He belonged to the Masons. I do not know much about them as a society, apart from the story of the secret handshake, but I know Granddad was a worshipful master in his day. After Mum was left to face the world on her own she would go to the Masonic meetings on a Thursday night with her affluent friends and she would enjoy their company with her one penny in her purse. Mum was the prime example of 'You don't have to be posh to be privileged.' Janine, Helen and I all wore long beautiful dresses when Mum was worshipful master for her year, and for that night my mum was a queen.

Granddad went every year to a health spa in Hertfordshire in a tiny village called Tring, and in 2004 I stood in the same tiny village and waved goodbye to my thirteen-year-old daughter, who spent the next three years at dance school there. The Royal Masonic Trust for Girls and Boys supported Lisa's vocational training with a financial donation – because of Granddad's connections we managed to get funding.

Thank you, Granddad Rose. Your legacy helped my talented daughter achieve her dream to train as a dancer.

Lisa never cried. From the day we left her she adapted to life away, but without fail, on chemo or not, I would travel to Tring and get her home for the weekend. We missed her, but I have no regrets about making that decision; and after a successful first year I fought hard for scholarships to keep her there. Lisa away at school finally gave me the freedom to concentrate on my own career, and I did get the promotion I applied for. I was given great responsibilities in the NHS, and I thrived on the challenge.

Ali and I lived happily in a trendy rented apartment in the centre of town, in walking distance of everywhere for both of us. We led a quiet, unassuming lifestyle and we were happy. The flat was a haven for Ali and his friends, and I loved the modern, low-maintenance living. I worked thirty hours a week, finishing early on a Friday. Then I would set off to pick Lisa up. Sometimes I would travel to the school and we would just spend the day together in Oxford. I would be back to work on Monday, and go salsa-dancing without fail on Monday evening. I joined the local gym and swam every morning. My fitness levels were improving fast. It was the best I had felt, physically, mentally and emotionally, for at least the last five years.

This life lasted exactly twelve months. In October 2005, when I was taking a shower, I found the lump, and from that day life changed for ever. On the hour I found that lump in 2005 I waved goodbye with regret to the sublime life I had built, and I saw it dismantled brick by brick with each hurdle of life over the next five years altering from sublime to ridiculous.

I am on the train returning home from London. Lisa and I have had a great time and the most significant thing I have gained from this two days is a contented reassurance that Lisa is now comfortable in her own life and capable of following her own life path. In fact for most of the two days she carried me. There were quiet times, but the silences were from contentment and, on my part, reflection about the wonderful memories that Lisa's nineteen years have given to me. I stare at this woman opposite me on the Tube, and she seems at home in the adult hub of London. Maybe she herself will be living here after uni, and maybe not. Lisa's choices are now only in Lisa's hands.

Me – Yes, Sharon Rose Who HAD Cancer in 2005 – the Here and Now, 22 February 2011

For four years after the cancer treatment I remained single. The difference was that I was a single parent too. But the single phenomenon faded into insignificance and I became happy in my own company. My fear of being alone faded into contentment. An elderly relative of mine pointed out that her life was a cul-de-sac compared to mine, which reminded her of Spaghetti Junction, and we laughed at this analogy.

We may be privileged enough to have a soulmate whilst on this earth, but some of us may not meet our soulmate in this life. Karmic soulmates are those who appear briefly in your life, carry you through traumas, laugh with you through the good times and remain in your life within your soul for ever. Chris was to become a karmic soulmate, but that's another story.

In March 2010 my first book was published, followed in 2011 by my second book, *Living in Grief, Loving in Grief*. Now I hope to have my third book published to inspire other women. Five years on I am still here. I didn't have a crystal ball to work with, and it took time for me to refocus my life in a positive way, but I did not waste any time. I move on now to deal with issues that come across my path of life. Should I have reconstruction? Should I not? These are questions still to be answered. Life is never on hold while we are on this earth.

I am back from the hospital appointment breathing a sigh of relief. I have come back to my husband, whose smiling face brightens my day. I walk in to a cuddle from a granddaughter I love. My daughter comes home from university and gives me a hug. Fiona doesn't give me a hug – just a glance tells me she loves me.

I read my emails and I open one from a fellow survivor I met in London.

'Hi, I've just read your book you wrote, which you kindly gave to each of us girls taking part in CRUK race for life the musical. I was so touched by your honesty of the journey you and many cancer survivors like us have travelled. Many pages of your book made me laugh out loud and yes . . . many were read though floods of tears! I could relate to the point you made about not making plans for the future as since my own cancer diagnosis in Autumn 2008, that's something I've never been able to do due to the uncertainty of time scales, a cancer diagnosis gives you. But after spending time with you and the girls this week but also your book . . . now I see a future and will MAKE FUTURE PLANS in my life! My Life restarts right now thanks to you Sharon. You are a lovely woman. X'

This is where I leave my story, and I go forward to my next check-up with these words imprinted in my heart. I have reached one person and helped her – someone I met for one day. These are the words I have waited for since the day I published my book. I am rich with happiness.

I am rich with happiness,
My life is sublime.
The ridiculous gave me strength
To see through the dark clouds
And see the sun shine.

To all who know me and supported me, love life, live life, celebrate the gift of life.